LESS THAN 1200 CALORIE DIET COOKBOOK

Dr. Kimberly Carlos

TABLE OF CONTENT

INTRODUCTION 7

CHAPTER ONE 9

Following a Diet Of Fewer Than 1200 Calories with Benefits 9

CHAPTER TWO 13

14-Day Meal Plan With Fewer Than 1200 Calories 13

Day 1: 13

Day 2: 13

Day 3: 14

Day 4: 14

Day 5: 15

Day 6: 15

Day 7: 16

Day 8: 16

Day 9: 17

Day 10: 17

Day 11: 18

Day 12: 18

Day 13: 19

Day 14: 19

CHAPTER THREE 21

Less than 1200 Calorie Diet Breakfast Recipes............ 21

1. Greek Yogurt Parfait.................................... 21

2. Veggie Omelette 22

3. Overnight Chia Pudding 23

4. Banana and Almond Butter Toast 24

5. Smoothie Bowl.. 24

6. Avocado and Tomato Toast 25

7. Berry and Spinach Smoothie 26

8. Cottage Cheese and Fruit Salad 27

9. Peanut Butter and Banana Wrap 28

10. Berry Breakfast Quinoa 29

Less than 1200 Calorie Diet Lunch Recipes................ 30

1. Grilled Chicken Salad.................................. 30

2. Quinoa and Black Bean Bowl.................................. 31

3. Spinach and Feta Stuffed Chicken Breast 32

4. Chickpea Salad with Lemon-Tahini Dressing 33

5. Tuna Salad Lettuce Wraps 34

6. Lentil Soup 34

7. Turkey and Avocado Lettuce Wraps 35

8. Caprese Salad 36

9. Zucchini Noodles with Pesto 37

10. Baked Sweet Potato and Chickpea Bowl 38

CHAPTER FOUR 39

Less than 1200 Calorie Diet Dinner Recipes 39

1. Grilled Salmon with Asparagus 39

2. Stir-Fried Tofu with Broccoli 40

3. Baked Chicken Breast with Roasted Brussels Sprouts
.... 41

4. Spaghetti Squash with Marinara Sauce 42

5. Veggie Stir-Fry with Brown Rice 43

6. Shrimp and Broccoli Quinoa Bowl 44

7. Baked Cod with Lemon and Herbs 45

8. Eggplant and Chickpea Curry 46

9. Turkey and Sweet Potato Skillet 47

10. Vegetable and Tofu Stir-Fry with Brown Rice 48

Less than 1200 Calorie Diet Snacks Recipes 49

1. Greek Yogurt and Berry Parfait 49

2. Sliced Cucumber with Hummus 50

3. Almond Butter and Banana Slices 51

4. Cottage Cheese with Pineapple 51

5. Apple Slices with Peanut Butter 52

6. Mixed Nuts 53

7. Sliced Bell Peppers with Guacamole 53

8. Carrot Sticks with Tzatziki Sauce 54

9. Edamame 54

10. Sliced Pear with Cottage Cheese 55

CONCLUSION 56

INTRODUCTION

Sarah had always struggled with her weight, and after years of fad diets and disappointment, she decided it was time for a change. She knew she needed something sustainable, something that wouldn't leave her feeling deprived. That's when she discovered the world of 1200-calorie diet recipes.

With determination in her heart, Sarah began exploring different low-calorie recipes. She scoured cookbooks, websites, and even joined an online community of like-minded individuals on a similar journey. Her goal was clear: to create delicious, filling meals that would fit within her daily 1200-calorie limit.

Sarah's mornings started with a hearty bowl of oatmeal topped with fresh berries and a sprinkle of almonds. For lunch, she enjoyed a colorful salad filled with crisp vegetables, lean protein, and a zesty vinaigrette. In the afternoon, she satisfied her snack cravings with yogurt and a handful of crunchy carrot sticks.

Dinner was where Sarah got creative. She experimented with various cuisines, tweaking recipes to make them lower in calories without sacrificing flavor.

Her favorite was a flavorful stir-fry loaded with colorful vegetables and tender strips of chicken, all seasoned with a tantalizing blend of herbs and spices.

As the weeks passed, Sarah noticed the pounds gradually melting away. She felt more energetic, and her clothes started fitting better. Her newfound love for cooking had not only transformed her body but also her relationship with food. Instead of viewing meals as indulgence, she saw them as an opportunity to nourish her body with wholesome, tasty dishes.

Sarah's journey with her 1200-calorie diet recipes was more than just a diet; it was a lifestyle change. She learned the art of portion control, discovered new ingredients, and developed a passion for cooking that she never knew existed. Most importantly, she found a way to enjoy food while still maintaining a calorie-conscious lifestyle.

With each passing day, Sarah's story became an inspiration to those around her. She showed them that a 1200-calorie diet didn't have to be a sentence of bland, unsatisfying meals. Instead, it could be a delicious journey towards a healthier, happier life.

CHAPTER ONE

Following a Diet Of Fewer Than 1200 Calories with Benefits

Following a diet of fewer than 1200 calories a day can be beneficial to some individuals, but it's important to do it safely and under the guidance of a healthcare professional, especially if you have specific health conditions or goals. Here's a general guideline on how to follow a diet with fewer than 1200 calories a day with potential benefits:

1. Consult a Healthcare Professional: Before starting any calorie-restricted diet, consult with a registered dietitian or healthcare provider to ensure it's appropriate for your individual needs and goals. They can help you determine the right calorie level and provide personalized guidance.

2. Set Clear Goals: Define your reasons for wanting to follow a calorie-restricted diet. It might be for weight loss, managing a medical condition, or improving overall health. Setting clear, realistic goals will help you stay motivated.

3. Calculate Your Calorie Needs: Use a reputable online calculator or consult with a dietitian to determine your daily calorie needs based on factors like age, gender, activity level, and weight goals. Ensure the calorie target is appropriate for your specific needs and goals.

4. Choose Nutrient-Dense Foods: Focus on nutrient-dense foods that provide essential vitamins, minerals, and fiber without excess calories. Include plenty of fruits, vegetables, lean proteins, whole grains, and healthy fats in your diet.

5. Portion Control: Pay attention to portion sizes to stay within your calorie limit. Measuring your food and using smaller plates can help with portion control.

6. Plan Balanced Meals: Plan meals that include a balance of protein, complex carbohydrates, and healthy fats. This balance can help you feel satisfied and maintain muscle mass while losing weight.

7. Stay Hydrated: Drink plenty of water throughout the day to stay hydrated and help control hunger. Sometimes, thirst is mistaken for hunger.

8. Monitor Your Progress: Keep a food diary or use a calorie-tracking app to monitor your daily intake and ensure you stay within your calorie limit.

This can help you identify areas for improvement.

9. Include Regular Exercise: Incorporate regular physical activity into your routine to support weight loss and overall health. Consult with a fitness professional to create an exercise plan that aligns with your calorie goals.

10. Listen to Your Body: Pay attention to hunger and fullness cues. Eating mindfully and slowly can help you recognize when you're truly hungry and when you've had enough.

11. Get Adequate Sleep: Ensure you're getting enough quality sleep, as sleep can affect hunger hormones and overall well-being.

12. Monitor Health Metrics: Regularly check in with your healthcare provider to monitor your progress, especially if you have specific health goals or conditions.

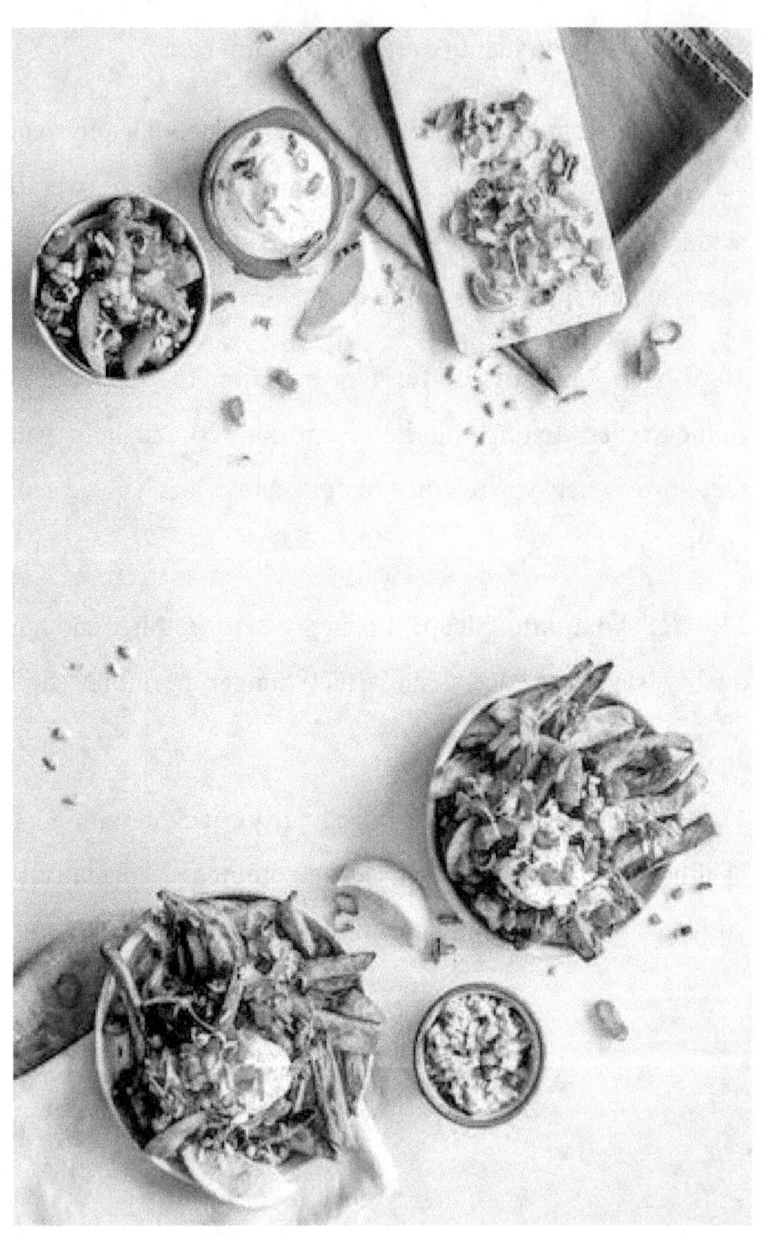

CHAPTER TWO

14-Day Meal Plan With Fewer Than 1200 Calories

Day 1:

- **Breakfast:** Scrambled eggs with spinach and tomatoes (200 calories)
- **Snack:** Greek yogurt with honey (100 calories)
- **Lunch:** Grilled chicken breast with mixed greens and balsamic vinaigrette (300 calories)
- **Snack:** Sliced cucumber with hummus (100 calories)
- **Dinner:** Baked salmon with quinoa and steamed broccoli (400 calories)

Day 2:

- **Breakfast:** Oatmeal with berries and a sprinkle of almonds (250 calories)
- **Snack:** Apple slices with peanut butter (150 calories)
- **Lunch:** Turkey and avocado lettuce wraps (300 calories)
- **Snack:** Carrot sticks with tzatziki sauce (100 calories)

- **Dinner:** Stir-fried tofu with mixed vegetables and brown rice (400 calories)

Day 3:

- **Breakfast:** Greek yogurt parfait with granola and berries (300 calories)
- **Snack:** Celery sticks with almond butter (150 calories)
- **Lunch:** Quinoa salad with chickpeas, cucumber, and lemon-tahini dressing (350 calories)
- **Snack:** Mixed nuts (100 calories)
- **Dinner:** Grilled shrimp with asparagus and a side salad (400 calories)

Day 4:

- **Breakfast:** Scrambled egg whites with spinach and mushrooms (200 calories)
- **Snack:** Cottage cheese with pineapple (150 calories)
- **Lunch:** Lentil soup with a side of mixed greens (350 calories)
- **Snack:** Sliced bell peppers with guacamole (100 calories)
- **Dinner:** Baked chicken breast with sweet potato and steamed green beans (400 calories)

Day 5:

- **Breakfast:** Smoothie with spinach, banana, almond milk, and protein powder (250 calories)
- **Snack:** Sliced pear with cottage cheese (150 calories)
- **Lunch:** Quinoa and black bean bowl with salsa and avocado (350 calories)
- **Snack:** Edamame (100 calories)
- **Dinner:** Broiled cod with quinoa and roasted Brussels sprouts (400 calories)

Day 6:

- **Breakfast:** Greek yogurt parfait with granola and mixed berries (300 calories)
- **Snack:** Sliced cucumber with hummus (100 calories)
- **Lunch:** Turkey and avocado lettuce wraps (300 calories)
- **Snack:** Mixed nuts (150 calories)
- **Dinner:** Grilled salmon with quinoa and steamed broccoli (400 calories)

Day 7:

- **Breakfast:** Scrambled egg whites with spinach and tomatoes (200 calories)
- **Snack:** Sliced apple with peanut butter (150 calories)
- **Lunch:** Chickpea salad with mixed greens and lemon-tahini dressing (350 calories)
- **Snack:** Carrot sticks with tzatziki sauce (100 calories)
- **Dinner:** Stir-fried tofu with mixed vegetables and brown rice (400 calories)

Day 8:

- **Breakfast:** Scrambled egg whites with spinach and mushrooms (200 calories)
- **Snack:** Sliced pear with cottage cheese (150 calories)
- **Lunch:** Lentil soup with a side of mixed greens (350 calories)
- **Snack:** Sliced bell peppers with guacamole (100 calories)
- **Dinner:** Baked chicken breast with sweet potato and steamed green beans (400 calories)

Day 9:

- **Breakfast:** Smoothie with spinach, banana, almond milk, and protein powder (250 calories)
- **Snack:** Mixed nuts (150 calories)
- **Lunch:** Quinoa and black bean bowl with salsa and avocado (350 calories)
- **Snack:** Edamame (100 calories)
- **Dinner:** Broiled cod with quinoa and roasted Brussels sprouts (400 calories)

Day 10:

- **Breakfast:** Greek yogurt parfait with granola and mixed berries (300 calories)
- **Snack:** Sliced cucumber with hummus (100 calories)
- **Lunch:** Turkey and avocado lettuce wraps (300 calories)
- **Snack:** Mixed nuts (150 calories)
- **Dinner:** Grilled salmon with quinoa and steamed broccoli (400 calories)

Day 11:

- **Breakfast:** Scrambled egg whites with spinach and tomatoes (200 calories)
- **Snack:** Sliced apple with peanut butter (150 calories)
- **Lunch:** Chickpea salad with mixed greens and lemon-tahini dressing (350 calories)
- **Snack:** Carrot sticks with tzatziki sauce (100 calories)
- **Dinner:** Stir-fried tofu with mixed vegetables and brown rice (400 calories)

Day 12:

- **Breakfast:** Greek yogurt with honey and a sprinkle of sliced almonds (250 calories)
- **Snack:** Celery sticks with peanut butter (150 calories)
- **Lunch:** Turkey and avocado lettuce wraps (300 calories)
- **Snack:** Sliced bell peppers with hummus (100 calories)
- **Dinner:** Grilled chicken breast with quinoa and steamed broccoli (400 calories)

Day 13:

- **Breakfast:** Scrambled egg whites with spinach and mushrooms (200 calories)
- **Snack:** Sliced pear with cottage cheese (150 calories)
- **Lunch:** Lentil soup with a side of mixed greens (350 calories)
- **Snack:** Carrot sticks with tzatziki sauce (100 calories)
- **Dinner:** Baked salmon with sweet potato and asparagus (400 calories)

Day 14:

- **Breakfast:** Smoothie with spinach, banana, almond milk, and protein powder (250 calories)
- **Snack:** Mixed nuts (150 calories)
- **Lunch:** Quinoa and black bean bowl with salsa and avocado (350 calories)
- **Snack:** Edamame (100 calories)
- **Dinner:** Broiled cod with quinoa and roasted Brussels sprouts (400 calories)

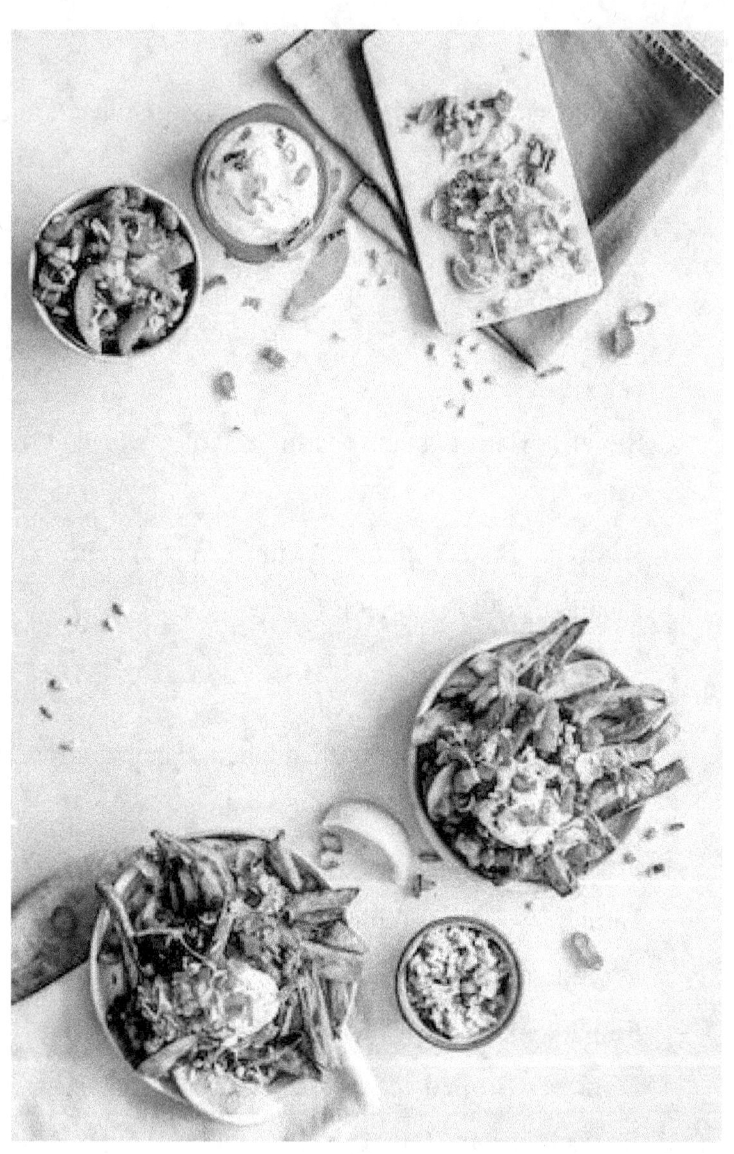

CHAPTER THREE

Less than 1200 Calorie Diet Breakfast Recipes

1. Greek Yogurt Parfait

Start your day with a protein-packed and satisfying Greek yogurt parfait topped with fresh fruits and crunchy granola.

Ingredients:

- 1/2 cup Greek yogurt
- 1/2 cup mixed berries (strawberries, blueberries, raspberries)
- 1/4 cup granola
- 1 teaspoon honey (optional)

Instructions:

1. In a glass or bowl, layer Greek yogurt at the bottom.

2. Add mixed berries on top of the yogurt.

3. Sprinkle granola over the berries.

4. Drizzle honey for extra sweetness if desired.

Cooking Time: 5 minutes

2. Veggie Omelette

Create a nutrient-packed omelette filled with colorful vegetables to kickstart your morning.

Ingredients:

- 2 large eggs
- 1/4 cup diced bell peppers (red, green, yellow)
- 1/4 cup diced tomatoes
- 1/4 cup diced onions
- Salt and pepper to taste
- Cooking spray or a teaspoon of olive oil for the pan

Instructions:

1. In a bowl, whisk the eggs, salt, and pepper.

2. Heat a non-stick skillet over medium-high heat and coat it with cooking spray or a touch of olive oil.

3. Pour the egg mixture into the skillet.

4. Add the diced vegetables evenly over one half of the omelette.

5. When the eggs are set but slightly runny on top, fold the omelette in half.

6. Cook for another minute or until it's fully set.

Cooking Time: 10 minutes

3. Overnight Chia Pudding

This make-ahead breakfast is not only low in calories but also packed with fiber and healthy fats.

Ingredients:

- 2 tablespoons chia seeds
- 1/2 cup unsweetened almond milk
- 1/2 teaspoon vanilla extract
- Fresh berries for topping (optional)

Instructions:

1. In a jar or bowl, mix chia seeds, almond milk, and vanilla extract.

2. Stir well and refrigerate overnight (or at least 4 hours).

3. In the morning, top with fresh berries if desired.

Cooking Time: 5 minutes (plus overnight refrigeration)

4. Banana and Almond Butter Toast

A simple, quick, and satisfying breakfast that combines the creaminess of almond butter with the natural sweetness of bananas.

Ingredients:

- 1 slice whole-grain bread
- 1 tablespoon almond butter
- 1/2 banana, thinly sliced

Instructions:

1. Toast the whole-grain bread until crispy.

2. Spread almond butter on the toasted bread.

3. Arrange banana slices on top.

Cooking Time: 5 minutes

5. Smoothie Bowl

A smoothie bowl is a fun and nutritious way to start your day, and you can customize it with your favorite toppings.

Ingredients:

- 1 cup unsweetened almond milk
- 1/2 frozen banana
- 1/2 cup frozen berries (strawberries, blueberries, or raspberries)
- 1 tablespoon chia seeds
- Toppings (e.g., sliced fruits, nuts, seeds, shredded coconut)

Instructions:

1. Blend almond milk, frozen banana, frozen berries, and chia seeds until smooth.

2. Pour the smoothie into a bowl.

3. Add your favorite toppings for texture and flavor.

Cooking Time: 5 minutes

6. Avocado and Tomato Toast

A savory and creamy breakfast toast topped with the goodness of avocado and ripe tomatoes.

Ingredients:

- 1 slice whole-grain bread
- 1/2 ripe avocado
- 1 small tomato, sliced
- Salt, pepper, and a pinch of red pepper flakes (optional)

Instructions:

1. Toast the whole-grain bread until crispy.

2. Mash the ripe avocado and spread it on the toasted bread.

3. Layer tomato slices on top.

4. Season with salt, pepper, and red pepper flakes if desired.

Cooking Time: 5 minutes

7. Berry and Spinach Smoothie

This green smoothie is a nutritious blend of leafy greens and sweet berries.

Ingredients:

- 1 cup unsweetened almond milk

- 1 cup fresh spinach leaves
- 1/2 cup mixed berries (strawberries, blueberries, raspberries)
- 1/2 banana
- 1 tablespoon honey (optional)

Instructions:

1. Blend almond milk, fresh spinach, mixed berries, banana, and honey (if using) until smooth.

2. Pour into a glass and enjoy.

Cooking Time: 5 minutes

8. Cottage Cheese and Fruit Salad

A protein-rich breakfast salad featuring creamy cottage cheese and fresh fruits.

Ingredients:

- 1/2 cup low-fat cottage cheese
- 1/2 cup mixed fresh fruits (e.g., pineapple, melon, berries)
- A drizzle of honey (optional)
- A sprinkle of chopped mint leaves (optional)

Instructions:

1. In a bowl, combine cottage cheese and mixed fruits.

2. Drizzle with honey and sprinkle with chopped mint leaves if desired.

Cooking Time: 5 minutes

9. Peanut Butter and Banana Wrap

A quick and satisfying breakfast wrap combining the creaminess of peanut butter with sliced bananas.

Ingredients:

- 1 whole-grain tortilla
- 2 tablespoons peanut butter (or almond butter)
- 1/2 banana, thinly sliced
- A sprinkle of cinnamon (optional)

Instructions:

1. Spread peanut butter evenly on the whole-grain tortilla.

2. Arrange banana slices on top.

3. Sprinkle with cinnamon if desired.

4. Roll up the tortilla and slice it in half.

Cooking Time: 5 minutes

10. Berry Breakfast Quinoa

Quinoa for breakfast? Absolutely! This protein-packed grain pairs perfectly with sweet berries.

Ingredients:

- 1/2 cup cooked quinoa (prepared according to package instructions)
- 1/2 cup mixed berries (strawberries, blueberries, raspberries)
- 1 tablespoon honey (optional)
- A sprinkle of chopped nuts (e.g., almonds, walnuts)

Instructions:

1. Cook quinoa according to package instructions.

2. In a bowl, mix cooked quinoa with mixed berries.

3. Drizzle with honey and sprinkle with chopped nuts if desired.

Cooking Time: 15 minutes (includes quinoa cooking time)

Less than 1200 Calorie Diet Lunch Recipes

1. Grilled Chicken Salad

Enjoy a light and protein-packed salad with tender grilled chicken and a variety of fresh vegetables.

Ingredients:

- 4 oz grilled chicken breast
- Mixed greens (lettuce, spinach, arugula)
- Cherry tomatoes
- Cucumber slices
- Red onion slices
- Balsamic vinaigrette dressing

Instructions:

1. Grill the chicken breast until cooked through (usually 15-20 minutes).

2. Let the chicken cool, then slice it.

3. Assemble a salad with mixed greens, cherry tomatoes, cucumber slices, red onion slices, and the sliced grilled chicken.

4. Drizzle with balsamic vinaigrette dressing.

Cooking Time: 20-25 minutes

2. Quinoa and Black Bean Bowl

A satisfying and fiber-rich bowl featuring quinoa, black beans, and colorful veggies.

Ingredients:

- 1/2 cup cooked quinoa
- 1/2 cup black beans (canned, rinsed and drained)
- Bell peppers (red, yellow, green)
- Corn kernels (cooked or canned)
- Avocado slices
- Lime juice
- Cilantro leaves

Instructions:

1. Cook quinoa according to package instructions.

2. In a bowl, combine cooked quinoa, black beans, bell peppers, corn kernels, and avocado slices.

3. Drizzle with lime juice and garnish with cilantro leaves.

Cooking Time: 15-20 minutes (includes quinoa cooking time)

3. Spinach and Feta Stuffed Chicken Breast

Delight in a flavorful and protein-packed stuffed chicken breast with spinach and feta cheese.

Ingredients:

- 4 oz boneless, skinless chicken breast
- 1 cup fresh spinach leaves
- 2 tablespoons crumbled feta cheese
- Olive oil
- Salt and pepper to taste

Instructions:

1. Preheat the oven to 375°F (190°C).

2. Butterfly the chicken breast.

3. Stuff the chicken with fresh spinach leaves and crumbled feta cheese.

4. Season with salt and pepper.

5. Heat olive oil in an oven-safe skillet over medium-high heat.

6. Sear the chicken on both sides until golden brown.

7. Transfer the skillet to the oven and bake for about 15 minutes or until the chicken is cooked through.

Cooking Time: 20-25 minutes

4. Chickpea Salad with Lemon-Tahini Dressing

This refreshing salad combines protein-rich chickpeas with a zesty lemon-tahini dressing.

Ingredients:

- 1 cup canned chickpeas (rinsed and drained)
- Mixed greens
- Cucumber slices
- Red onion slices
- Cherry tomatoes
- Lemon-tahini dressing (blend tahini, lemon juice, garlic, and water)

Instructions:

1. Combine chickpeas, mixed greens, cucumber slices, red onion slices, and cherry tomatoes in a bowl.

2. Drizzle with lemon-tahini dressing.

Cooking Time: 10 minutes

5. Tuna Salad Lettuce Wraps

Swap out traditional bread for lettuce leaves in this light and protein-packed tuna salad.

Ingredients:

- 1 can of tuna in water, drained
- Greek yogurt (as a mayo substitute)
- Diced celery
- Diced red bell pepper
- Lettuce leaves (e.g., iceberg or Romaine)

Instructions:

1. In a bowl, mix the drained tuna, Greek yogurt, diced celery, and diced red bell pepper.

2. Spoon the tuna salad into lettuce leaves to create wraps.

Cooking Time: 10 minutes

6. Lentil Soup

Warm up with a hearty and nutritious lentil soup that's full of fiber and plant-based protein.

Ingredients:

-   1 cup dry green or brown lentils
-   Chopped carrots, celery, and onion
-   Vegetable broth
-   Herbs and spices (e.g., thyme, bay leaves, garlic powder)

Instructions:

1. Rinse the lentils thoroughly.

2. In a large pot, sauté chopped carrots, celery, and onion until softened.

3. Add rinsed lentils, vegetable broth, and herbs and spices.

4. Simmer until lentils are tender (usually 30-40 minutes).

Cooking Time: 40-50 minutes

7. Turkey and Avocado Lettuce Wraps

Enjoy these low-carb and high-protein lettuce wraps filled with lean turkey and creamy avocado.

Ingredients:

- Lean ground turkey
- Lettuce leaves
- Sliced avocado
- Salsa

Instructions:

1. Cook the lean ground turkey until browned.

2. Spoon the cooked turkey into lettuce leaves.

3. Top with sliced avocado and salsa.

Cooking Time: 15 minutes

8. Caprese Salad

Savor the classic flavors of Italy in a simple and fresh Caprese salad.

Ingredients:

- Fresh mozzarella cheese
- Ripe tomatoes
- Fresh basil leaves
- Balsamic glaze or vinegar

- Olive oil
- Salt and pepper

Instructions:

1. Slice the fresh mozzarella cheese, ripe tomatoes, and fresh basil leaves.

2. Arrange the slices on a plate, alternating cheese, tomatoes, and basil.

3. Drizzle with balsamic glaze or vinegar, olive oil, and season with salt and pepper.

Cooking Time: 10 minutes

9. Zucchini Noodles with Pesto

Enjoy a low-calorie and low-carb lunch with zucchini noodles tossed in vibrant pesto sauce.

Ingredients:

- Zucchini noodles (zoodles)
- Pesto sauce (homemade or store-bought)
- Cherry tomatoes
- Pine nuts (optional)

Instructions:

1. Cook the zucchini noodles according to package instructions (usually a quick sauté).

2. Toss the cooked zoodles with pesto sauce.

3. Add halved cherry tomatoes and pine nuts (if desired).

Cooking Time: 10 minutes

10. Baked Sweet Potato and Chickpea Bowl

A satisfying and fiber-rich bowl featuring baked sweet potatoes, chickpeas, and an array of colorful veggies.

Ingredients:

- 1 medium sweet potato, diced
- 1/2 cup canned chickpeas (rinsed and drained)
- Mixed greens
- Bell pepper strips
- Red onion slices
- Tahini dressing (mix tahini, lemon juice, and water)

Instructions:

1. Preheat the oven to 400°F (200°C).

2. Toss diced sweet potato and chickpeas with olive oil, salt, and pepper.

3. Roast in the oven until sweet potatoes are tender (usually 20-25 minutes).

4. Assemble a bowl with mixed greens, roasted sweet potato, chickpeas, bell pepper strips, and red onion slices.

5. Drizzle with tahini dressing.

Cooking Time: 25-30 minutes

CHAPTER FOUR

Less than 1200 Calorie Diet Dinner Recipes

1. Grilled Salmon with Asparagus

This dinner features a healthy and flavorful grilled salmon fillet paired with roasted asparagus.

Ingredients:

- 4 oz salmon fillet
- Fresh asparagus spears
- Olive oil
- Lemon slices
- Salt and pepper

Instructions:

1. Preheat the grill to medium-high heat.

2. Season the salmon with olive oil, lemon slices, salt, and pepper.

3. Grill the salmon for about 4-5 minutes per side or until it flakes easily.

4. Toss asparagus with olive oil, salt, and pepper, then roast in the oven at 400°F (200°C) for 10-15 minutes.

Cooking Time: 20-25 minutes

2. Stir-Fried Tofu with Broccoli

A quick and satisfying stir-fry with tofu and broccoli in a savory sauce.

Ingredients:

- Firm tofu, cubed
- Broccoli florets
- Soy sauce
- Garlic and ginger, minced
- Sesame oil
- Red pepper flakes (optional)

Instructions:

1. In a wok or large skillet, heat sesame oil over medium-high heat.

2. Add minced garlic and ginger and stir-fry for a minute.

3. Add cubed tofu and cook until golden brown.

4. Add broccoli florets and soy sauce. Stir-fry until broccoli is tender.

5. Optionally, sprinkle with red pepper flakes for heat.

Cooking Time: 20-25 minutes

3. Baked Chicken Breast with Roasted Brussels Sprouts

A simple yet delicious dinner featuring baked chicken breast and crispy roasted Brussels sprouts.

Ingredients:

- Boneless, skinless chicken breast
- Brussels sprouts, trimmed and halved
- Olive oil
- Garlic powder
- Paprika
- Salt and pepper

Instructions:

1. Preheat the oven to 375°F (190°C).

2. Season the chicken breast with olive oil, garlic powder, paprika, salt, and pepper.

3. Place the chicken on one side of a baking sheet.

4. Toss Brussels sprouts with olive oil, salt, and pepper on the other side of the baking sheet.

5. Bake for about 25-30 minutes or until the chicken is cooked through and Brussels sprouts are crispy.

Cooking Time: 30-35 minutes

4. Spaghetti Squash with Marinara Sauce

Enjoy a low-carb alternative to traditional pasta with spaghetti squash and marinara sauce.

Ingredients:

- Spaghetti squash
- Marinara sauce (store-bought or homemade)
- Fresh basil leaves
- Parmesan cheese (optional)

Instructions:

1. Preheat the oven to 375°F (190°C).

2. Cut the spaghetti squash in half lengthwise and remove seeds.

3. Place squash halves cut side down on a baking sheet and

roast for about 30-40 minutes.

4. Scrape the squash with a fork to create "noodles."

5. Top with marinara sauce, fresh basil leaves, and Parmesan cheese if desired.

Cooking Time: 40-45 minutes

5. Veggie Stir-Fry with Brown Rice

A colorful and nutrient-rich vegetable stir-fry served with wholesome brown rice.

Ingredients:

- Mixed vegetables (bell peppers, broccoli, carrots, snap peas)
- Firm tofu or chicken (optional)
- Brown rice, cooked
- Stir-fry sauce (soy sauce, ginger, garlic, sesame oil)

Instructions:

1. Heat olive oil in a wok or large skillet over high heat.

2. Add tofu or chicken (if using) and cook until browned.

3. Add mixed vegetables and stir-fry for a few minutes until they start to soften.

4. Pour in stir-fry sauce and continue to cook until the vegetables are tender.

5. Serve over cooked brown rice.

Cooking Time: 20-25 minutes

6. Shrimp and Broccoli Quinoa Bowl

A protein-packed and nutritious bowl featuring succulent shrimp, quinoa, and tender broccoli.

Ingredients:

- Shrimp, peeled and deveined

- Quinoa, cooked

- Broccoli florets

- Olive oil

- Lemon juice

- Garlic, minced

- Red pepper flakes (optional)

Instructions:

1. In a large skillet, heat olive oil over medium-high heat.

2. Add minced garlic and red pepper flakes (if using) and cook for a minute.

3. Add shrimp and cook until pink and opaque.

4. Toss in cooked quinoa and steamed broccoli florets.

5. Drizzle with lemon juice.

Cooking Time: 20-25 minutes

7. Baked Cod with Lemon and Herbs

A light and flavorful dinner featuring baked cod with a zesty lemon and herb marinade.

Ingredients:

- Cod fillet
- Lemon juice and zest
- Fresh herbs (e.g., parsley, thyme)
- Olive oil
- Garlic, minced
- Salt and pepper

Instructions:

1. Preheat the oven to 375°F (190°C).

2. Mix lemon juice, lemon zest, minced garlic, olive oil, and fresh herbs.

3. Place the cod fillet on a baking sheet, season with salt and pepper, and drizzle the lemon-herb mixture over it.

4. Bake for about 15-20 minutes or until the fish flakes easily.

Cooking Time: 15-20 minutes

8. Eggplant and Chickpea Curry

A satisfying and flavorful vegetarian curry with eggplant, chickpeas, and aromatic spices.

Ingredients:

- Eggplant, diced
- Chickpeas (canned, rinsed and drained)
- Curry paste or powder
- Coconut milk
- Fresh cilantro leaves

- Cooked rice (brown or white)

Instructions:

1. Heat olive oil in a large pot or skillet.

2. Add diced eggplant and cook until it starts to soften.

3. Stir in curry paste or powder and cook for a minute.

4. Add chickpeas and coconut milk. Simmer until the eggplant is tender and the flavors meld.

5. Serve over cooked rice and garnish with fresh cilantro leaves.

Cooking Time: 25-30 minutes

9. Turkey and Sweet Potato Skillet

A one-pan wonder featuring lean ground turkey and sweet potatoes in a flavorful and satisfying dish.

Ingredients:

- Lean ground turkey
- Sweet potatoes, diced
- Onion, chopped

- Garlic, minced

- Spinach leaves

- Paprika, cumin, and chili powder

- Olive oil

- Salt and pepper

Instructions:

1. Heat olive oil in a large skillet.

2. Add chopped onion and garlic and sauté until fragrant.

3. Add ground turkey, sweet potatoes, and spices. Cook until turkey is browned and sweet potatoes are tender.

4. Stir in spinach leaves until wilted.

Cooking Time: 25-30 minutes

10. Vegetable and Tofu Stir-Fry with Brown Rice

A plant-based stir-fry with tofu and an array of colorful vegetables served over wholesome brown rice.

Ingredients:

- Firm tofu, cubed

- Mixed vegetables (bell peppers, broccoli, carrots, snow peas)
- Brown rice, cooked
- Stir-fry sauce (soy sauce, ginger, garlic, sesame oil)

Instructions:

1. Heat olive oil in a wok or large skillet over high heat.

2. Add tofu and cook until golden brown.

3. Add mixed vegetables and stir-fry until tender-crisp.

4. Pour in stir-fry sauce and continue cooking until heated through.

5. Serve over cooked brown rice.

Cooking Time: 20-25 minutes

Less than 1200 Calorie Diet Snacks Recipes

1. Greek Yogurt and Berry Parfait

Indulge in a creamy and fruity parfait that's high in protein and low in calories.

Ingredients:

- 1/2 cup Greek yogurt
- Mixed berries (strawberries, blueberries, raspberries)
- Honey (optional)

Instructions:

1. In a glass or bowl, layer Greek yogurt.

2. Add a generous portion of mixed berries.

3. Drizzle with honey for extra sweetness if desired.

Preparation Time: 5 minutes

2. Sliced Cucumber with Hummus

A refreshing and crunchy snack featuring cucumber slices and creamy hummus.

Ingredients:

- Cucumber, thinly sliced
- Hummus (store-bought or homemade)

Instructions:

1. Arrange the cucumber slices on a plate.

2. Dip them in hummus and enjoy.

Preparation Time: 5 minutes

3. Almond Butter and Banana Slices

This quick and satisfying snack combines the richness of almond butter with the natural sweetness of bananas.

Ingredients:

- Banana, thinly sliced
- Almond butter (or peanut butter)

Instructions:

1. Spread almond butter on banana slices.

2. Enjoy this creamy and fruity snack.

Preparation Time: 5 minutes

4. Cottage Cheese with Pineapple

A protein-packed and sweet snack that combines creamy cottage cheese with juicy pineapple.

Ingredients:

- Low-fat cottage cheese

- Fresh pineapple chunks (or canned in juice, drained)

Instructions:

1. In a bowl, combine cottage cheese and pineapple chunks.

2. Enjoy this high-protein, low-calorie treat.

Preparation Time: 5 minutes

5. Apple Slices with Peanut Butter

A classic snack pairing sweet apple slices with creamy peanut butter for a satisfying crunch.

Ingredients:

- Apple, thinly sliced
- Peanut butter (or almond butter)

Instructions:

1. Dip apple slices in peanut butter.

2. Savor the delicious contrast of sweet and savory.

Preparation Time: 5 minutes

6. Mixed Nuts

A simple and nutritious snack that provides healthy fats, protein, and a satisfying crunch.

Ingredients:

Mixed nuts (e.g., almonds, walnuts, cashews)

Instructions:

1. Measure out a portion of mixed nuts.

2. Enjoy this on-the-go snack that's rich in nutrients.

Preparation Time: Instant

7. Sliced Bell Peppers with Guacamole

A colorful and tasty snack pairing bell pepper strips with creamy guacamole.

Ingredients:

- Bell peppers (various colors), sliced
- Guacamole (store-bought or homemade)

Instructions:

1. Dip bell pepper strips in guacamole.

2. Enjoy this combination of crispness and creaminess.

Preparation Time: 5 minutes

8. Carrot Sticks with Tzatziki Sauce

A refreshing and low-calorie snack featuring carrot sticks and tangy tzatziki sauce.

Ingredients:

- Carrot sticks
- Tzatziki sauce (store-bought or homemade)

Instructions:

1. Dip carrot sticks into tzatziki sauce.

2. Savor the crunchy and creamy flavors.

Preparation Time: 5 minutes

9. Edamame

Edamame is a protein-rich and satisfying snack that's quick and easy to prepare.

Ingredients:

Edamame (frozen or fresh)

Instructions:

1. Steam or boil edamame until tender (usually 4-5 minutes for frozen).

2. Sprinkle with a touch of sea salt if desired.

3. Enjoy these tasty soybean pods as a snack.

Preparation Time: 5-7 minutes

10. Sliced Pear with Cottage Cheese

A delightful combination of sweet and creamy featuring sliced pears and cottage cheese.

Ingredients:

- Ripe pear, thinly sliced
- Low-fat cottage cheese

Instructions:

1. Arrange pear slices on a plate.

2. Serve with a side of cottage cheese for a creamy contrast.

Preparation Time: 5 minutes

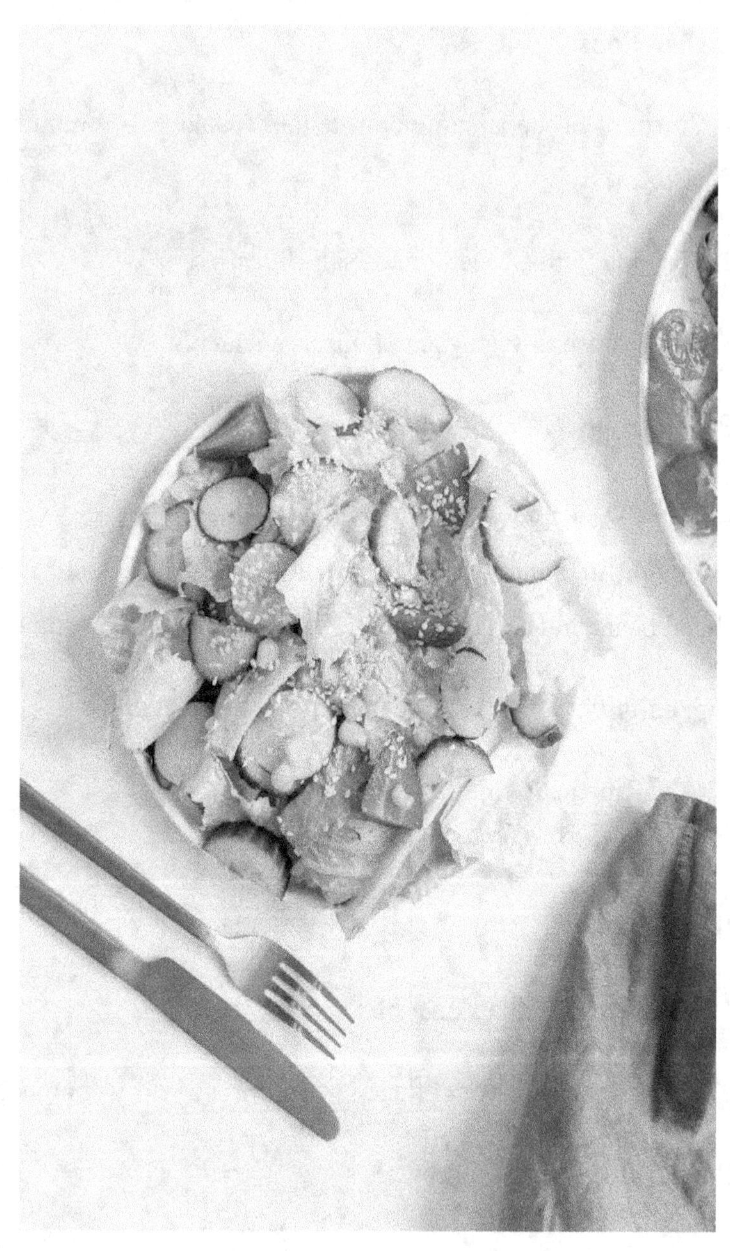

CONCLUSION

A less than 1200 calorie diet can be an effective approach for those seeking weight loss, managing specific health conditions, or simply adopting a healthier lifestyle.

Throughout this dietary regimen, we have explored various aspects, from meal planning to recipes, in an effort to provide a comprehensive understanding of its benefits and considerations.

First and foremost, it's important to recognize that a diet restricted to fewer than 1200 calories per day should be undertaken with caution and under the guidance of a healthcare professional or registered dietitian.

It is not suitable for everyone, and individual needs vary based on factors such as age, gender, activity level, and overall health.

One of the key benefits of such a diet is its potential for effective weight management. By creating a calorie deficit, the body can tap into stored fat for energy, ultimately leading to weight loss. Additionally, this approach can encourage portion control, mindful eating, and a greater focus on nutrient-dense foods, which can be valuable habits for long-term health.

However, it's crucial to strike a balance and prioritize nutrient quality over calorie quantity. Emphasizing whole foods, lean proteins, ample fruits and vegetables, and healthy fats is essential to ensure that your body receives the necessary vitamins, minerals, and macronutrients for optimal function.

Nevertheless, the less than 1200 calorie diet should not be considered a quick fix or a sustainable long-term solution.

Extreme calorie restriction can lead to nutrient deficiencies, muscle loss, and other health issues. It is crucial to monitor your progress, stay hydrated, and listen to your body's hunger and fullness cues.

In summary, this dietary regimen can be a useful tool for those with certain medical conditions, like obesity or type 2 diabetes, when supervised by a healthcare professional. It may help improve blood sugar control and reduce the risk of related complications.